Table of Contents

Introduction 4

What is a kidney stone? 5

Are all kidney stones the same? 5

What is the most important factor to prevent kidney stone formation? 5

What kind of diet plan is recommended to prevent stones? 6

Will it help or hurt to take a vitamin or mineral supplement? 9

    General Recommendations 11

Lifestyle Tips For Kidneystone 13

    Food and drinks to avoid on a kidney stone diet 14

Takeaway 17

Kidney Stone Diet Recipes 17

    Juice - Cucumber Mint Cooler 17

    Almond crusted Tilapia 18

    Turkey Taco Salad 19

    Kidney Bean Salad 20

    Tangy Crunchy Kidney Bean Salad 21

    Rajma 22

    Chicken Caprese with Tomato-Basil Cream 23

Skinny Pizza Margherita 25

Spicy Stone Fruit Salsa 26

Jamaican jerk chicken 27

5-4-3-2-1 biscuits 29

Oatmeal Chocolate Chip/Raisin Cookies 30

Philly steak roll 31

Chocolate chip oatmeal cookies 32

Angel's Whole Wheat Pizza Crust 33

Cheese Pizza 34

Krista's Breakfast Cookies 35

Fajita Pizza 36

Chicken and Veggies with Red Kidney Beans 39

Taco Soup 40

Chili 41

Kidney Bean Pasta (UK measures) 42

Chicken Chili 43

Tofu Chili 44

Red Beans & Rice 46

Salsa Bean Salad 48

Hurry-up fill-me-up burritos 49

beef chilli 50

Pasta Fagiole 51

Kidney disease diet Sample Meal Plan 52

    Kidney diet menu: Day 1... 52

    Kidney diet menu: Day 2... 54

    Kidney diet menu: Day 3... 56

Tips for a kidney stone diet 58

Conclusion 59

Introduction

Kidney stones in the urinary tract are formed in several ways. Calcium can combine with chemicals, such as oxalate or phosphorous, in the urine. This can happen if these substances become so concentrated that they solidify. Kidney stones can also be caused by a buildup of uric acid. Uric acid buildup is caused by the metabolism of protein. Your urinary tract wasn't designed to expel solid matter, so it's no surprise that kidney stones are very painful to pass. Luckily, they can usually be avoided through diet.

Did you know that 1 in 10 people will have a kidney stone over the course of a lifetime? Recent studies have shown that kidney stone rates are on the rise across the country.\

If you have kidney stones, you may need to follow a special diet plan. First, your healthcare professional will run blood and urine tests to find out what kind of risk factors you may have. Then your healthcare professional will tell you the diet changes and medical treatment you need to prevent having kidney stones come back.

A registered kidney dietitian can help you make the necessary changes in your diet plan and lifestyle.

What is a kidney stone?
A kidney stone is a hard mass that forms from crystals in the urine. For most people, natural chemicals in the urine keep stones from forming and causing problems.

Are all kidney stones the same?
No. The most common types of kidney stones are calcium stones followed by uric acid stones. Diet changes and medical treatment are individualized based on the type of stone, to prevent them from coming back.

What is the most important factor to prevent kidney stone formation?
One of the best things you can do to avoid kidney stones is to drink plenty of water every day. This will help make sure that you urinate frequently to avoid any build up of calcium or uric acid.

Don't underestimate your sweat! Saunas, hot yoga and heavy exercise may sound good for your health, but they also may lead to kidney stones. Why? Loss of water through sweating whether due to these activities or just the heat of summer may lead to less urine production. The more you sweat, the less you will urinate, which allows stone-causing minerals to settle and deposit in the kidneys and urinary tract.

Hydrate with water. Be sure to keep well hydrated, especially when doing exercise or activities that cause a lot of sweating. You should drink 2-3 quarts of liquid or 8-12 cups per day to produce a good amount of urine. Try to avoid sodas (especially those with high amounts of fructose), sweetened iced tea and grape fruit juice.

What kind of diet plan is recommended to prevent stones?
There is no single diet plan for stone prevention. Most diet recommendations are based on stone types and individualized for each person.

1. Calcium Oxalate Stones: most common stones

Oxalate is naturally found in many foods, including fruits and vegetables, nuts and seeds, grains, legumes, and even chocolate and tea. Some examples of foods that have high levels of oxalate include peanuts, rhubarb, spinach, beets, Swiss chard, chocolate and sweet potatoes. Limiting intake of these foods may be beneficial for people who form calcium oxalate stones which is the leading type of kidney stone.

Eat and drink calcium foods such as milk, yogurt, ice cream and some cheese and oxalate-rich foods together during a meal. The oxalate and calcium from the foods are more likely to bind to one another in the stomach and intestines before entering the kidneys. This will make it less likely that kidney stones will form.

Calcium is not the enemy but it tends to get a bad rap!This is most likely due to its name and misunderstanding that calcium is the main cause in calcium-oxalate stones. A diet low in calcium actually increases your chances of developing kidney stones.

Don't reduce the calcium in your diet. Work to cut back on the sodium in your diet and to pair calcium-rich foods with oxalate-rich foods. The recommended calcium intake to prevent calcium stones is 1000-1200 mg per day (you can eat 3 servings of dairy products with meals to meet the recommendation).

Extra sodium causes you to lose more calcium in your urine.Sodium and calcium share the same transport in the kidney so if you eat high sodium foods it will increase calcium leakage in the urine. Therefore, a high sodium diet can increase your chances for developing another stone. There are many sources of "hidden" sodium such as canned or commercially processed foods as well as restaurant-prepared and fast foods.

You can lower your sodium intake by choosing fresh low sodium foods which can help to lower calcium leakage in the urine and will also help with blood pressure control if you have high blood pressure.

2. Uric acid stones: another common stone

Red meat, organ meats, and shellfish have high amounts of a natural chemical compound known as purines. High purine intake leads to a higher production of uric acid and a larger acid load for the kidneys to excrete. Higher uric acid excretion leads to more acidic urine. The high acid concentration of the urine makes it easier for uric acid stones to form.

To prevent uric acid stones, cut down on high-purine foods such as red meat, organ meats, beer/alcoholic beverages, meat-based gravies, sardines, anchovies and shellfish. Follow a healthy diet plan that has mostly vegetables and fruits, whole grains, and low-fat dairy products. Limit sugar-sweetened foods and drinks, especially those that have high fructose corn syrup. Limit alcohol because it can increase uric acid levels in the blood and avoid short term diets for the same reason. Decreasing animal-based protein and

Will it help or hurt to take a vitamin or mineral supplement?

The B vitamins which include thiamine, riboflavin, niacin, B6 and B12 have not been shown to be harmful to people with kidney stones. In fact, some studies have shown that B6 may actually help people with high urine oxalate. However, it is best to check with your healthcare professional or dietitian for advice on the use of vitamin C, vitamin D, fish liver oils or other mineral supplements containing calcium since some supplements can increase the chances of stone formation in some individuals.

Is there anything else to do to help prevent kidney stones?

1. It's Not "One and Done." Passing a kidney stone is often described as one of the most painful experiences

an individual will experience. Unfortunately, it's not always a one-time event. Take action NOW! Without the right medicines, diet, and fluid intake, stones can come back. Returning kidney stones could also mean there are other problems, including kidney disease.

2. When Life Hands You Kidney Stones... don't worry. And as the saying goes, "make lemonade out of lemons." It's important to think about diet changes along with prescription medicines. While it may seem easier to just take a pill to fix a medical problem, consider what lifestyle changes will also make a difference for your health

Next time you drive past a lemonade (or limeade) stand, consider your kidneys. Chronic kidney stones are often treated with potassium citrate, but studies have shown that limeade, lemonade and other fruits and juices high in natural citrate may offer the same stone-preventing benefits. Beware of the sugar, though, because it may increase kidney stone risk. Instead, buy sugar-free lemonade, or make your own by mixing lime or lemon juice with water and using a sugar substitute if needed. Adding 3 tablespoons of fresh lemon juice per one quart of water will help you lower kidney stone formation.

Although grapefruit is citrus it may have a bad effect on kidney stones therefore it is not recommended.

General Recommendations
Drink plenty of fluid: 2-3 quarts/day

This includes any type of fluid such as water, coffee and lemonade which have been shown to have a beneficial effect with the exception of grapefruit juice and soda.

This will help produce less concentrated urine and ensure a good urine volume of at least 2.5L/day

Limit foods with high oxalate content

Spinach, many berries, chocolate, wheat bran, nuts, beets, tea and rhubarb should be eliminated from your diet intake

Eat enough dietary calcium

Three servings of dairy per day will help lower the risk of calcium stone formation. Eat with meals.

Avoid extra calcium supplements

Calcium supplements should be individualized by your physician and registered kidney dietitian

Eat a moderate amount of protein

High protein intakes will cause the kidneys to excrete more calcium therefore this may cause more stones to form in the kidney

Avoid high salt intake

High sodium intake increases calcium in the urine which increases the chances of developing stones

Low salt diet is also important to control blood pressure.

Avoid high doses of vitamin C supplements

It is recommend to take 60mg/day of vitamin C based on the US Dietary Reference Intake

Excess amounts of 1000mg/day or more may produce more oxalate in the body

Lifestyle Tips For Kidneystone
Stay hydrated

Fluids, especially water, help to dilute the chemicals that form stones. Try to drink at least 12 glasses of water a day.

Up your citrus intake

Citrus fruit, and their juice, can help reduce or block the formation of stones due to naturally occurring citrate. Good sources of citrus include lemons, oranges, and grapefruit.

Eat lots of calcium (and vitamin D)

If your calcium intake is low, oxalate levels may rise. It's preferable to get your calcium from food, rather than from supplements, as these have been linked to kidney stone formation. Good sources of calcium include milk, yogurt, cottage cheese, and other types of cheeses. Vegetarian sources of calcium include legumes, calcium-set tofu, dark green vegetables, nuts, seeds, and blackstrap molasses. If you don't like the taste of cow's milk, or, if it doesn't agree with you, try lactose-free milk, fortified soy milk, or goat's milk. Also make sure to include foods high in vitamin D each day. Vitamin D helps the body absorb more calcium. Many foods are fortified with this vitamin. It's also found in fatty fishes, such as salmon, egg yolks, and cheese.

Food and drinks to avoid on a kidney stone diet
Limit salt

High sodium levels in the body, can promote calcium buildup in urine. Avoid adding salt to food, and check the labels on processed foods to see how much sodium they contain. Fast food can be high in sodium, but so can regular restaurant food. When you're able, ask that no salt be added to whatever you order on a menu. Also, take note of what you drink. Some vegetable juices are high in sodium.

Lower your animal protein intake

Many sources of protein, such as red meat, pork, chicken, poultry, fish, and eggs, increase the amount of uric acid you produce. Eating large amounts of protein also reduces a chemical in urine called citrate. Citrate's job is to prevent the formation of kidney stones.

Alternatives to animal protein include quinoa, tofu (bean curd), hummus, chia seeds, and Greek yogurt. Since protein is important for overall health, discuss how much you should eat daily with your doctor.

A plant-based diet may be ideal

Eat oxalates wisely. Foods high in this chemical may increase formation of kidney stones. If you've already had kidney stones, you may wish to reduce or eliminate oxalates from your diet completely. If you're trying to avoid kidney stones, check with your doctor to determine if limiting these foods is enough. If you do eat foods containing oxalates, always make sure to eat or drink a calcium source with them. This will help the oxalate bind to the calcium during digestion, before it can reach your kidneys. Foods high in oxalate include:

chocolate

beets

nuts

tea

rhubarb

spinach

swiss chard

sweet potatoes

Don't drink colas

Avoid cola drinks. Cola is high in phosphate, another chemical which can promote the formation of kidney stones.

Reduce or eliminate added sugar intake

Added sugars are sugars and syrups that are added to processed foods and drinks. Added sucrose and added fructose may increase your risk of kidney stones. Keep an eye on the amount of sugar you eat, in processed foods, such as cake, in fruit, in soft drinks, and in juices. Other common added sugar names include corn syrup, crystallized fructose, honey, agave nectar, brown rice syrup, and cane sugar.

Takeaway

Kidney stones are typically a painful condition. Fortunately, diet can be an effective tool in managing and preventing kidney stones. Staying hydrated and avoiding certain foods that are high in salt and sugar, and pairing calcium with oxalate rich foods are important elements of a kidney stone diet.

Kidney Stone Diet Recipes

Juice - Cucumber Mint Cooler

Ingredients

2 medium cucumbers

2 stalks celery

1 small handful fresh mint, plus additional for garnish

2 limes, outer peel cut away and discarded

Directions

1. Run all ingrediants through a juicer

2. Pour over ice and garnish with mint spigs

Cucumbers are hydrating and cooling, and a good diuretic. They help to flush wastes through the kidneys and dissolve uric acid accumulates such as kidney and bladder stones. Celery also contains a lot of natural sodium to help keep you hydrated.

Almond crusted Tilapia

Ingredients

4 Tilapia fillets

4 Tbsp Fat Free Mayo

2 Tbs Honey

3 tsp Mustard - any kind, I prefer stone ground or brown.

1/2 Cup Almonds, ground

Directions

Mix Mayo, honey and mustard.

Place tilapia in pan coated with cooking spray.

Spread half of the mayo mixture over the tilapia.

Sprinkle half of the almonds on top and pat down into the mayo.

Flip fillets over and cover with remaining mayo mixture and almonds

bake at 350 for 15 minutes.

Turkey Taco Salad
Ingredients

2 oz ground turkey

1 1/2 cups romaine lettuce

1/4 cup red kidney beans

1/4 cup cheddar cheese

1/8 cup onions

1/2 oz tortilla chips

2 tbsp salsa

Directions

Brown turkey and then add the taco seasoning.

Chop lettuce and add kidney beans and onion. Rinse the lettuce, onion and kidney beans.

Add the turkey and cheese to the salad.

Crush tortilla chips and add to the top of the salad.

Add salsa and enjoy!

Kidney Bean Salad
Ingredients

1 serving dark red kidney beans

4 tbsp fat free mayonnaise

2 tbsp fat free sour cream

1/3 cup celery, diced

2 tbsp onions, chopped

Directions

Rinse and drain the kidney beans.

Mix sour cream and mayo until smooth.

Mix kidney beans, celery, onions and dressing.

Refrigerate for several hours before serving.

Tangy Crunchy Kidney Bean Salad

Ingredients

2 large celery stalks, diced

1 can (8 oz) sliced water chestnuts, drained

1 can (27 oz) dark red kidney beans, drained

2 hard boiled eggs, diced

1 Tbsp finely diced raw onion

2 Tbsp vinegar

2 Tbsp Sugar equivalent (Splenda or Equal)

1 Tbsp yellow mustard

1/4 cup Miracle Whip Free

Directions

Makes 6 one-cup servings

Drain cans of kidney beans & water chestnuts. Toss drained kidney beans, diced water chestnuts, chopped celery, finely chopped onion & hard boiled eggs in large bowl.

Blend vinegar, sugar substitute, mustard & Miracle Whip till smooth consistency. Toss salad with this dressing & serve. Can be made the day before.

Rajma

Ingredients

4 cups red kidney beans

1 cup raw onions, chopped

1 can crushed tomatoes

1 tbsp salt

1 tbsp pepper, red or cayenne

2 cups water

1 tbsp canola oil

Directions

Saute onions in oil until golden brown.

Add crushed tomatoes, cook for a few minutes.

Add kidney beans, water, salt, and pepper. Heat through. Serve alone or with basmati rice.

TIPS:

-Use canned kidney beans to make this quickly, be sure to rinse the beans before adding them.

-You can add as much or as little water to the pot depending on what consistency you like.

-You can also add garlic and or ginger to change up the flavors.

-If you REALLY want to change the flavor, buy MDH channa masala (in my opinion the best channa masala brand) or chat masala and add around 1/4 teaspoon to the dish.

Chicken Caprese with Tomato-Basil Cream
Ingredients

2/3 C. Seasoned Bread Crumbs

1/3 C. Parmesan cheese, grated

1 t. Dried Basil

1/4 t Salt

1/4 t Pepper

3 T. Olive oil

2 T. Lemon Juice

4 Skinned and boned chicken breast halves

Tomato-Basil Cream

1 C. Spaghetti sauce

1 t. Dried Basil

2 T. Light Sour Cream

Directions

To prepare the chicken for baking:

Stir together first 5 ingredients in a shallow bowl. Whisk together olive oil and lemon juice until blended. Dip chicken into olive oil mixture, and dredge in bread crumb mixture, pressing to coat.

Place in a lightly greased 11"x7" baking dish (I use a pizza stone). Spray top of the chicken with Pam when you place it in the baking dish or on the stone.

Bake at 375 degrees for 30 minutes or until chicken is done. Serve with Tomato-Basil Cream: garnish with lemon slices, Basil spirgs (if desired).

Skinny Pizza Margherita
Ingredients

1 recipe Quinoa-Flaxseed Pizza Dough

1 recipe Better-than-Pesto Puree

1 cup grape tomatoes, halved lengthwise

4 ounces soft goat cheese, crumbled

Directions

1. Raise the oven rack to the highest level, then preheat oven to 400° F. If using a pizza stone,

place it in the oven to preheat.

2. Place the dough on a pizza screen or preheated stone, spread with the pesto, then scatter the tomatoes and cheese across the top.

3. Bake until the dough is nicely browned and crispy, 18 to 20 minutes

Spicy Stone Fruit Salsa

Ingredients

4 peaches, chopped

2 cups cherries, pitted and chopped

2 small or 1 large jalapeno pepper, diced

1 lime, zested and juiced

Tips

Salsa simply means "sauce" in Spanish, and although we usually think of pico de gallo--that piquant combination of tomatoes, peppers, onions, and cilantro--as salsa, you can use any combination of fruits and vegetables.

Use any combination of fruits here: nectarines, plums, cherries, or peaches.

If you like a spicier salsa, leave the ribs and seeds in the peppers; if you don't like spice, remove them.

Directions

Combine all ingredients. Allow to rest at room temperature for 20 minutes before serving.

Makes 2 1/2 cups; 1/2 cup per serving

Jamaican jerk chicken
Ingredients

Serves 4

2 tbsp veg oil

2 tbsp plain flour

1 tbsp jamaican jerk seasoning

salt and black pepper

1 chisken, jointed into 8 pieces

225g Brown rice

400g can red kidney beans, rinsed and drained

50g butter

1 plantain, thinly sliced

Directions

preheat the oven to 200oC/Gas 6. Add the oil to a roasting pan.On a large plate, mix the flour with the jerk seasoning along with the salt and pepper. Add the 8 pieces of chicken and toss to coat.Place the chicken on the roasting pan and bake in the oven for 25-30 minutes. In the mean time, cook the brown rice in boiling, salted water for about 15 minutes or until tender, add the red kidney beans for the last 3-4 mins of cooking time.

About 10 minutes before the chicken is ready, melt the butter in a frying pan and fry the plantain slices, occasionally turning them over until brown and crispy. Drain on kitchen paper, serve with chicken, brown rice and kidney beans.

5-4-3-2-1 biscuits
Ingredients

5 tbs baking soda

4 half cup measures of whole wheat flour (2 cups)

3 half cup measures of white flour (1 1/2 cups)

2 pinches of salt (or use salted butter)

1 stick of butter

2 cups of milk (I use powdered made into milk right then)

Directions

Preheat oven to 450degrees

1. combine dry ingredients,

2. cut in butter (I use a kitchen aid flat blade for ease)

3. Mix in milk by hand

drop large tablespoon scoops onto baking stone (or sheet) -makes about 24

Cook for 10-15 minutes.

Oatmeal Chocolate Chip/Raisin Cookies
Ingredients

3/4 cup Smart Balance 50/50 butter blend or other butter

.5 cup sugar (or Splenda, which I used)

1 cup brown sugar

1 tsp cinnamon

1 tsp baking soda

1 cup flour

.5 raisins, can add up to 1 cup

.5 cup milk chocolate chips

3 cups plain instant oatmeal

1 egg

25 cup skim or 1% milk

1 tsp vanilla

Directions

Preheat oven to 350 degrees.

Put softened butter, egg, sugars, milk and vanilla into large bowl and beat until light and fluffy.

Combine flour, cinnamon, baking soda and salt in another bowl and add to butter mixture. Mix well.

Stir in oatmeal, raisins and chocolate chips.

Drop by rounded teaspoons onto greased cookie sheets or baking stone.

Bake 12-15 minutes, remove from cookie sheet and cool on wire racks.

Makes 4 dozen, 3 dozen if you use tablespoon sized dough balls.

Philly steak roll
Ingredients

7-8 oz shaed lean roast beef lunchmeat

8 slices 2% american cheese torn into strips

1 cup chopped onion (approx)

1 cup chopped green and/or red peppers (approx)

1 clove garlic

1 tsp oregano

1 small can or cup of mushrooms

2 pillsbury crusty french bread

Directions

chop up onion, peppers, mushrooms and some garlic and cook until tender crisp. Layer half meat, veggies and cheese & roll up. Put the other roll together and then connect them on stone. brush with egg & sprinkle with oregeno bake at 400.

Chocolate chip oatmeal cookies
Ingredients

1 1/4 c flour , 1 tsp baking soda , 1/2 tsp salt, 1 c butter, 3/4 C sugar, 2 eggs,

3/4 C packed brown sugar,

1 tsp vanilla extract, 3 Cup quick oats,

11 oz package of hershey's semi sweet chocolate chips

Directions

Preheat oven 375 degrees

put butter, eggs, vanilla, baking soda, salt, and sugars and beat well in mixing bowl, add flour, mix, add oats then add chocolate chips.

Drop by tablespoon onto baking stone or sheet

bake for 7-8 minutes take out of oven and cool on cooling rack YUM

makes 51 cookies

Angel's Whole Wheat Pizza Crust
Ingredients

2.5 cups whole wheat flour

2.5 tsp baking powder

1 tsp sea salt (or just plain salt)

1 tsp yeast (or more if you like the flavor of it)

3/4 cup water

1/4 cup olive oil

Directions

Mix dry ingredients, add wet, stir until ball forms

knead into stiff ball, roll out onto pizza pan or stone with a rolling pin or by hand. For thick crust makes one 16 inch pizza for a thinner crust makes 2 12 inch pizzas. Top with favorite sauce and toppings. Bake at 400 for 20-25 minutes.

Cheese Pizza
Ingredients

1 Moma Mary's Whole Wheat Thin & Crispy Pizza Crust

1 1/2 cups Classico Basil/Tomato Pasta Sauce

2 cups 2% Shredded Mozzarella

Directions

Preheat oven & pizza stone (if using) to 425*.

Spread pasta sauce over crust. Distribute cheese evenly over crust. Cook for 15 min or until cheese is melted.

Makes 8 Slices

Krista's Breakfast Cookies
Ingredients

1 cup old fashioned oats

1 cup skim milk powder

2 tbsp dried fruit (raisins, crasins, other) I used SunMaid Fruit Bits

2 tbsp bittersweet chocolate chips

1 cup unsweetened applesauce

1 tsp baking powder

3 tbsp whole wheat flour

1 packet sweetener (I used Purevia)

1/4 tsp salt

1 tsp cinnamon

Optional

2 tbsp PB2 powdered peanut butter (added in this version)

or

1 tbsp flaxseeds (not figured in this version for cal count)

Directions

Combine dry ingredients, mix thoroughly. Add applesauce and mix well. Form into 6 mounds on cookie sheet or baking stone. Can also be made in a bar pan or small baking pan. Bake at 350 for 15-20 minutes.

Fajita Pizza
Ingredients

1 Medium Green pepper

1 Medium Red Bell Pepper

1 Medium sweet onion

2 boneless, skinless chicken breast halves (about 4 oz)

2 packages (10 Ounce each) refridgerated Pizza Crust

1 teaspoon vegetable oil, divided

1 teaspoon chili powder

1/2 teaspoon ground cumin

1 garlic clove, pressed (or very finely chopped)

1/4 cup Thick and Chunky salsa (mild, medium or hot)

2 cups (8 Ounces) Mexican blend (Taco) shredded cheese, divided

2 Tablespoons snipped fresh cilantro

2 Fresh plum tomatos diced (optional)

Additional thick and chunky salsa and sour cream (optional)

Directions

1. Preheat oven to 425 degrees F. Cut bell peppers into 1/2-inch thick strips. Cut Onion into 1/2-inch-thick wedges. Cut Chicken crosswise into thin strips.

2) Lightly sprinkle Pizza Stone (or Pizza Pan) with flour, unroll both packages of pizza dough and arrange side by side on baking stone, shaping into a circle. Using lightly flouredrolling pin, roll dough to edge of baking stone, pressing seams to seal.

3) Heat Stir-Fry skillet over high heat. Add 1/2 teaspoon of the oil and chicken; stir fry 2-3 minutes until chicken is no longer pink. Remove from skillet. Add remaining oil, bell peppers, onion and seasoning mix to skillet. Press Garlic over vegetables using a garlic press, or add minced garliced to pan with vegetables. Stir-fry 1-2 mins or until vegetables are crisp-tender. Remove skillet from heat; stir in chicken and salsa.

4) Sprinkle half of the cheese evenly over crust, arrange chicken mixture over cheese, then spinkle remaining cheese over chicken mixture.

5) Bake 18-22 mins or until crust is golden brown. Remove from oven. Sprinkle cilantro over pizza ; let

stand 10 mins, cut into wedges. Serve with additional salsa and sour cream if desired.

Chicken and Veggies with Red Kidney Beans

Ingredients

3 - Chicken Breast, no skin or bone

1 can (10.75 oz) - Campbell's Cream of Mushroom condensed soup (Healthy Request)

1 cup - Light Red Kidney Beans

1 cup - Broccoli & Cauliflower, frozen

1 cup - Crinkle Cut Zuccini, frozen

2 cups - Water

1 - Slow Cooker or Crock Pot

Directions

Put all ingredients in slow cooker. Cook for 8 hours.

Taco Soup

Ingredients

1 lb. lean ground beef

1 14 oz. can tomato sauce

1 14 oz. can diced tomatos w/green chilies

1 4 oz. can chopped green chilies

2 cans corn

2 cans dark kidney beans

1 pkg. taco seasoning

Toppings (not included in nutrition info):

Frito chips

Fat-Free Cheese

Fat-Free Sour Cream

Directions

Brown ground beef over medium heat.

While cooking beef, simmer the following items on low heat in a large pot: tomato sauce, diced tomatos, green chilies, corn, kidney beans, and taco seasoning.

Add beef. Bring to boil, and then simmer for 15 more minutes.

Serve and enjoy. Garnish with chips, cheese, and sour cream!

Chili

Ingredients

1 tbls cayenne

1 tbls chili powder

1 cup chopped onion

1 cup chopped green pepper

2 tsp garlic

4 cups kidney beans

4 cups stewed tomotoes

1 lb ground beef, lean

Directions

brown ground beef, put in crockpot

saute the onion, garlic and green pepper, add to crockpot

add kidney beans and stewed tomatoes.

stir in seasonings

cook on low in crockpot for 6 hours.

you could add everything uncooked, but I'm leary of that with ground beef. and I like the flavor of the sauted onions, garlic and green bell pepper.

Kidney Bean Pasta (UK measures)
Ingredients

3.5 oz wholewheat penne pasta

400g can red kidney beans

400g can chopped tomatoes

1 tbsp ground turmeric

1 tsp freshly milled pepper

1 tsp cayenne pepper

Directions

Cook the pasta according to the instructions on the packet. (I do not add salt)

Drain and add back into the pan.

Add the canned tomatoes, drained kidney beans and seasonings.

Allow this to reduce over a low heat to the desired consistency.

Chicken Chili
Ingredients

2 lbs chicken breast

28 oz diced canned tomatoes

2-14.5 ounce kidney beans

2 cups onion diced

2 cups green pepers diced

1 tbsp chili powder

36 tsp old el paso taco seasoning

Directions

Place chicken, onion, green pepper and chili powder in slow cooker on high x 1 hour, then low x 4 hours.

Cut chicken into small pieces, add tomatoes, old el paso taco seasoning and kidney beans. Cook in slow cooker for additional 3 hours.

Dish up and serve.

Add low fat or no fat sour cream, low fat or no fat cheddar cheese or baked tositos. Not included in recipe.

Tofu Chili
Ingredients

Extra Firm Tofu - 3 blocks

Chili Beans - 2 cans

Kidney Beans - 2 cans

Diced Tomatos - 2 cans

Tomato Sauce - 1 can

Mixed Vegetables - 1 package (16 oz)

Taco Bell Taco Seasoning - 1 packet

Chili Powder - 3 TBS

Cumin - 1 TSP

Garlic Powder - 1 TSP

Onion Powder - 1 TSP

Directions

Drain (but don't squeeze) and crumble tofu into large stock pot.

Add chili beans, kidney beans, diced tomatos, tomato sauce and mixed vegetables. Stir together.

Add Taco Seasoning - Stir

Add Chili Powder - Stir

Add Cumin, Garlic and Onion - Stir

Cook on medium - high until it begins to boil

Reduce heat and simmer for 20 minutes, stirring occasionally to prevent burning on the bottom of the pot.

Great when served with crackers and shredded cheese!

Red Beans & Rice
Ingredients

1 large red onion, chopped

2 garlic cloves, minced

2 teaspoons olive oil

1 carrot, chopped

2 celery ribs, chopped (I omitted)

1 bell pepper, chopped (any color)

1 teaspoon oregano

1/4 teaspoon thyme

1 teaspoon basil

1 teaspoon marjoram

1/8 teaspoon crushed red pepper flakes

1 (28 ounce) can tomatoes

1 (15 ounce) can kidney beans, rinsed and drained

1 tablespoon deli prepared mustard or dijon-style mustard

1 tablespoon maple syrup or brown sugar

2 tablespoons fresh parsley, chopped

1/2 teaspoon salt

1/4 teaspoon pepper

Directions

In a soup pot, saute onions and garlic in oil until onions are tender.

Add the carrots, celery, bell pepper, oregano, thyme, basil, marjoram and crushed red-pepper. Cook over medium heat for 10 minutes, stirring occasionally.

Stir in the tomatoes, kidney beans, mustard, maple syrup and parsley. Simmer gently for 5 minutes.

Stir in salt and pepper.

Server as a soup in bowls or over rice.

Cooked rice for serving (4 cups) calculated in the calories. 1/2 cup per serving.

Salsa Bean Salad

Ingredients

Black Beans 1 cup

Dark Red Kidney Beans 1 cup

Corn 1 cup

Onions 1 cup

Green Peppers 1/2 cup

Tomatoes 1 cup

Cheese 1 cup

Salsa 12 tablespoons

Directions

Drain Black Beans , Kidney Beansand Corn.. Mix in a bowl with all remaining ingredients, Onions, Peppers,Cheese, Salsa, Tomatoes. Chill, and Enjoy. You can add more salsa to taste. Serves 4

Hurry-up fill-me-up burritos
Ingredients

*Brown Rice, long grain, 1 cup cooked

Heinz - dark red kidney beans, 1 can (398ml)

Yellow Sweet Corn, Frozen, 1 cup kernels

Salsa, .75 cup

casa mendosa tortillas- whole wheat, 10 serving

Cheddar Cheese, 1 cup, shredded (optional)

Directions

In a large skillet over medium heat combine

cooked rice

kidney beans rinsed & drained

corn

salsa

cook over medium heat for 3-4 min until warmed through

spoon mixture onto tortillas

sprinkle with cheese

roll up tortillas

makes 10 burritos

you can add anything else that you like in burritos

this is a great way to get rid of leftover rice

beef chilli
Ingredients

450g lean minced beef

400g can chopped tomatoes

400g can kidney beans

1cup chopped carrot

30g tomato paste

30g chilli paste

3 cloves garlic

Directions

serves four

brown beef in pan then add chilli, grlic and tomato paste, draind kidney beans add to pot with can of tomatoes, simmer for 20 mins

serve with rice or baked potato

Pasta Fagiole
Ingredients

3.5 cup whole tomatoes (1- 28 oz can, undrained), pureed

1 cup tomato sauce (1- 8 oz can)

1 cup water

1 medium onion, chopped

2 garlic cloves, minced

1 tbsp olive oil

1.5 tbsp parsely

1 dash salt

1 dash pepper

3.5 cups red kidney beans (2- 15.5 oz cans), drained and rinsed

Directions

Lightly brown onion and garlic in olive oil. Add pureed tomatoes, tomato sauce, and water (can add more or less water to make more or less "soupy"). Add parsely, salt, and pepper. Cover and cook 1 hour. Then, add drained and rinsed kidney beans. Uncover and cook 30 minutes more. Serve over Ditalini pasta with parmesan cheese.

Kidney disease diet Sample Meal Plan

Kidney diet menu: Day 1
Breakfast

Ziptop Omelet

English muffin or toasted bread

Jam or jelly, margarine or butter

Fresh grapes

Coffee or tea

Sweetener or creamer

Lunch

Blackened shrimp pineapple salad

Low-sodium crackers or crisp bread

Lemon cookies

Lemon-lime soda

Dinner

Stuffed green peppers

Dinner rolls

Margarine or butter

Stuffed strawberries

Sparkling water

Day 1 tips:

Adjust Ziptop Omelet recipe for the number of omelets you plan to serve. You can make extra to refrigerate for an even quicker breakfast the next day. Reheat in the microwave for 20 to 30 seconds.

Increase shrimp in the salad if you are on a higher protein diet. Use leftover shrimp to make shrimp spread with crackers for a snack.

Make lemon cookies and serve as dessert at lunch or for an in-between-meals snack.

Buy grapes to serve at breakfast—they can be used for the second day's salad and for the third day's dinner, dessert or snack.

Use the extra pineapple as a snack or a dessert if you have leftovers once you make the blackened shrimp pineapple salad.

Buy enough strawberries for the stuffed strawberries recipe, the second day's pancake recipe and snacks, if desired.

Leftover stuffed peppers are easy to refrigerate or freeze for a quick lunch or dinner later in the week.

Kidney diet menu: Day 2
Breakfast

Egg in a Hole

Homemade Pan Sausage

Toasted bread

Jam or jelly, margarine or butter

Pineapple juice

Lunch

Tuna veggie salad

Sliced bread or pita bread

Lemon cookies

Home-brewed iced tea with lemon and sweetener

Dinner

Slow rotisserie-style chicken

Red wine vinaigrette asparagus

Pasta tossed in olive oil and garlic

Chilled or frozen grapes

Decaffeinated coffee or herb tea

Day 2 tips:

Make a batch of Homemade Pan Sausage and freeze patties on waxed paper and place in a freezer bag. You can prepare individual servings quickly throughout the week.

Tuna veggie salad calls for steamed vegetables, but you can add uncooked veggies if desired.

Home-brewed iced tea tastes fresh and is free of phosphate additives compared to some canned or bottled prepared teas.

Use leftover chicken from dinner for third day's lunch salad.

Kidney diet menu: Day 3
Breakfast

Cottage cheese pancakes with fresh strawberries

Whipped topping or syrup

Scrambled egg or egg whites

Coffee or tea

Sweetener or creamer

Lunch

Lemon curry chicken salad

Naan (Indian flatbread) or pita bread

Cranberry juice

Dinner

Cilantro-lime cod

Lettuce, cucumber and carrot salad

Basic salad dressing

Steamed Rice

Luscious Lime Dessert

Lemon-lime soda

Day 3 tips:

Include the eggs if you need a higher protein breakfast. Use low-cholesterol eggs or egg whites only if you are concerned about cholesterol. Egg whites are very low in phosphorus.

If you have time, make the lemon curry chicken salad the evening before so flavors can blend together.

Look for fresh cod or any comparable white fish on sale this week. You can also use frozen cod, sole or halibut.

The basic salad dressing recipe has only one milligram of sodium for two tablespoons, compared to 250 to 400 mg for commercially prepared salad dressing. It will keep for several weeks in the refrigerator.

To jazz up steamed rice, add your favorite low-sodium herb seasoning blend. Make extra rice for a kidney-friendly fried rice dish later in the week.

Tips for a kidney stone diet

Having kidney stones increases your risk of getting them again unless you actively work to prevent them. This means taking medications prescribed to you for this purpose, and watching what you eat and drink.

If you currently have stones, your doctor will run diagnostic tests, to determine what type you have. They will then prescribe a specific diet plan for you, such as the DASH Diet. Tips that will help include:

drink at least twelve glasses of water daily

drink citrus juices, such as orange juice

eat a calcium-rich food at each meal, at least three times a day

limit your intake of animal protein

eat less salt, added sugar, and products containing high fructose corn syrup

avoid foods and drinks high in oxalates and phosphates

avoid eating or drinking anything which dehydrates you, such as alcohol.

Conclusion

The kidney-friendly foods above are excellent choices for people following a renal diet.

Remember to always discuss your food choices with your healthcare provider to ensure that you are following the best diet for your individual needs.

Dietary restrictions vary depending on the type and level of kidney damage, as well as the medical interventions in place, such as medications or dialysis treatment.

While following a renal diet can feel restrictive at times, there are plenty of delicious foods that fit into a healthy, well-balanced, kidney-friendly meal plan.

CKD is long-standing progressive decline in kidney health.

You can prevent or reduce some of the health complications of moderate to severe CKD by limiting the amount of protein, sodium, phosphorus, and potassium in your diet.

A registered dietitian can make individualized nutrition recommendations based on your specific needs and health status.

Remember that a number of factors influence the best type of kidney diet that someone can follow, including: the stage of their renal disease, type of treatment

they are on, and presence of other medical conditions.

Even though a healthy diet that is similar to the DASH diet or Mediterranean diet has been slow the progression of kidney disease and other diseases like heart disease too, some patients will still need to follow a special diet that is more restrictive. To be safe, always speak with your doctor before changing your diet, especially if you have chronic kidney disease. The DASH diet and Mediterranean diet are not intended for people on dialysis, who should work with a dietician to make sure they are managing their nutrient intake carefully.

We conclude that integrating dietary manipulations into a comprehensive strategy will help prevent or ameliorate complications of CKD including acidosis, hyperkalemia, hyperphosphatemia and uremic symptoms and possibly influence CKD progression. We believe particular attention should be paid. To correcting metabolic acidosis with either sodium bicarbonate supplements or more simply with diet instructions how to include supplements of fruits and vegetables and to lower the intake of sodium chloride as well as phosphates by choosing foods that provide low contents of these ions. Changing the diet by concentrating on these dietary constituents will allow us to maximize the renoprotective anti-proteinuric effect of renin angiotensin system blockers. These considerations on dietary approaches for CKD prevention and management are particularly valuable for low-resource setting worldwide where patients with CKD are beset with numerous challenges often traceable to poverty and a lack of access to life-saving dialysis and transplantation. The feasibility of these management approaches for CKD and its risk factors even in low-income countries is exemplified by the program set up in the communities of Eastern Nepal in collaboration with the International Society of Nephrology (ISN). Dietary recommendation of low-sodium intake and increase of fruits and vegetable together with low-cost anti-hypertensive, anti-diabetic or renoprotective drugs as deemed appropriate, have been able to control proteinuria and slow renal function decline in more than a third of 3,400 individuals on active monitoring.

Regarding the very low protein diet with essential keto acids and amino acids regimen, there is recent and reassuring evidence for its efficacy and nutritionally safety but efforts are needed to improve compliance with dietary regimens. Nutritional educational programs and dieticians could help to increase patient adherence to dietary recommendations. We also recommend that components of the diet and regular monitoring of nutritional status should be jointly assessed by physicians and dieticians, just as recommended for patients with inherited metabolic defects, cirrhosis and diabetes.

Made in the USA
Columbia, SC
01 August 2021